Live to *120*

Love Every Minute

Live to 120

Love Every Minute

JOEL E. REED

Live to 120

Published by Lucid Books in Brenham, TX.
www.LucidBooks.net

Scripture quotations taken from the New English Bible, Copyright © Cambridge University Press and Oxford University Press 1961, 1970.

First Printing 2012

ISBN-13: 978-1-935909-44-6
ISBN-10: 1935909444

CONTENTS

INTRODUCTION

D o you have any idea how much your actions can influence the rate at which you age? Read on and you will be surprised. Does the goal of reaching 120 seem unrealistic? It may be too conservative. But first, let's understand the process.

What is aging? It happens to all of us, but just what is going on? Is it inevitable? Can we slow down the process?

Just defining the word "aging" is a challenge. What do we really mean when we refer to aging? It isn't as simple as it sounds. My wife used to ask the question, "Are we really getting old?" Then she would say that all she had to do was look in the mirror and she could see the telltale signs. She referred to the graying hair, the wrinkles, the brown spots, the thinning skin and all the things we quickly recognize as a sign that one is, indeed, getting older. Defining it, though, is something like the dilemma that Supreme Court Justice Potter Stewart faced when trying to define pornography in a case before court. He said, "I know it when I see it."

But is this a normal process related to our genes or is it the result of wear and tear and residuals of diseases and injuries? Is it related to diet with too much or too little food? Did we not get enough vitamins or minerals in our diet or too much fat and cholesterol? Did we fail to exercise enough?

To begin to understand aging, we must first explore what is really going on. Are genes responsible for the different rates of aging we see in our friends and neighbors, or are there other factors at play? Why do some parts of our bodies age and fail earlier than others?

The bottom line remains: what causes aging and can we do anything about it? Can we avoid failure of some of our bodily functions? Hopefully we can get a better understanding of the processes and our part in controlling them.

There are vast differences in how fast different people age. I looked around the room at a recent meeting and recognized a friend who I knew to be over 90 years of age. He was engaged in an animated conversation and would move about the room erect and with a strong gait. I am sure that anyone who did not know his age would have guessed that he was no older than 75. In the same room was a friend twenty years younger than the other who was bent over, hobbling along on a walker. Why such a great difference? Was one blessed with good genes and the other with bad ones? Or had one been the victim of several debilitating diseases and the other not? Is it a combination of these factors?

The perplexity remains. What are its causes and can we do anything about it? Can we slow it down? Can we avoid the loss of some of our bodily functions?

Hopefully we can get a better understanding of the process and our part in controlling it.

Let us explore the important factors.

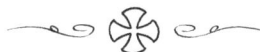

IS IT YOUR GENES?

G enes play an important part, at least in setting the stage for what is possible. Look at the species differences in average age. A mayfly is born, lives, reproduces and dies in about 1 day, a dog about 14 years, and a giant sequoia tree over 2000 years (the oldest known one estimated at 3500 years). What do our genes say is a life expectancy? Most scientists estimate that to be around 120 years, maybe more. Why don't we live up to that potential?

Lets look at historical life expectancies.

Bronze age	(2000-3000 BC)	18 years
Classic Greece	(300-500 BC)	20-30 years
Early 20th century	(1900-1910)	30-40 years
Current world average		70 years
U.S. Average	(50th in world)	78.37 years
The principality of Monaco	(1st in world)	89.73 years

What has caused this dramatic change? Note that most of the change has been in the last 100 years. Have our genes suddenly changed? Not likely. The process of evolution is a slow process with changes in small increments over hundreds of years,

The genes haven't changed that much in all those years. A treasure trove of information was obtained about our ancestry with the discovery of Ötzi, the "ice man" in 1991 in the Italian alps. Because of where he died, protected from the crushing weight of the glacier and frozen continuously, his remains could be studied in great detail. He lived 5300 years ago. A forensic restoration was made in the same manner that law enforcement restores the appearance of a corpse with proven uncanny accuracy. Look at the forensic restoration of Ötzi in James M. Deem's Mummy Tombs by going to YouTube and searching for "Ötzi the iceman". I think you will agree that he could walk by you on the street today and you would not notice anything unusual. It is clear that our genes are changing very slowly and cannot account for our rapidly increasing longevity in this last century.

Remember too that all genes are not good genes. Only a couple have been discovered that enhance longevity and more than a thousand have been identified that are related to diseases that may shorten our lives. Research is currently being conducted on the genome of people who have lived to very old age to see if there is a genetic key to resisting disease but there has been no conclusive evidence yet.

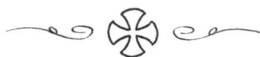

IS IT THE ENVIRONMENT?

M an had little control over the environment until the 20th century. Worldwide plagues and epidemics had tremendous negative effects on great populations. Though great pandemics are still possible (some say it is just a matter of time), they are more likely to be limited to a single continent, country or village. Injuries which we consider minor today often became infected in earlier centuries and led to an early death. Water sources were often contaminated and spread serious and fatal diseases. Disposal of waste was primitive if at all. This continues today in parts of the world.

Great epidemics spread rapidly and affected entire populations. The great influenza epidemic of 1918-1919 killed somewhere between twenty and forty million and is considered the most lethal epidemic of all time. In one year it killed more than the Bubonic plague in four years. Even today, the annual influenza epidemic which occurs each winter causes twenty to forty thousand excess deaths in the United States alone. The great Bubonic plague of the thirteenth and fourteenth centuries is one example. It wiped out one third of the people in Europe and perhaps more in Asia. Other examples include the cholera pandemic of 1817-1823, numerous epidemics in various parts of the world, the current AIDS epidemic, and many epidemics of yellow fever. Currently the ongoing epidemics of malaria in Africa and other parts of the world kills nearly a million victims each year. Perhaps sanitation has more to do with the prevention of disease and early death than medicine. Clean water supplies are essential. Sewers to carry away and treat human waste have been important in the prevention of diarrheal diseases. Immunization prevents many infectious diseases that used to threaten entire populations. For example, smallpox has been completely eradicated from the earth in our time because of vaccination. Below are listed examples of infections which we can now prevent or treat with a high rate of success. The following can be prevented or modified by immunization:

Measles
Mumps
Chickenpox
Diphtheria
Pertussis (Whooping cough)
German Measles
Tetanus
Hepatitis A & B
Influenza
Haemophilus influenzae
Pneumococcus infections
Meningococcal infections

Polio
Rabies
Rotavirus
Shingles
Human papilloma virus (Cancer of the cervix)

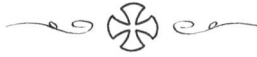

IS THERE PLANNED OBSOLESCENCE?

TELOMERASE THEORY

Telomeres are the tails or tips of the chromosomes. They seem to protect the DNA of the chromosome from damage but shorten each time the cell reproduces. The shorter they become, the more likely damage may occur to the chromosome. Telomeres resist shortening in cells which produce telomerase. Normal body cells which produce telomerase are those which have a short life cycle and must reproduce frequently. Examples are white blood cells, which last only a week or so, and red blood cells, which last about four months. Telomeres have been lengthened experimentally with increased longevity but the other side of the equation is that one of the factors allowing cancer cells to grow uninhibited is their ability to form telomerase. Much research remains to be done before we can apply this to humans but it raises great hopes.

IMMUNOLOGICAL THEORY

Our immune system gradually declines with age. Weakness or loss of immunologic protection from infections caused by bacteria, viruses, fungi or inactivation of toxins and even identification and destruction of foreign cells (cancer) leaves us more susceptible to these damaging conditions.

HORMONAL THEORY

Some changes in hormone levels are obvious and symptomatic, such as what women note when they are menopausal. Most, however, are insidious such as gradual loss of bone mass, change in muscle to fat ratio, and decreasing libido. Hormone replacement therapy can change many of those effects. Estrogen, either from natural or synthetic sources. has been used to counteract the symptoms of the menopause for generations. Beyond symptomatic relief, actual physical benefits have been observed such as delaying the loss of bone substance, improved appearance of the skin, improved vaginal lubrication, and even slowing of the atrophy (shrinkage) of the cells of the vaginal wall. Human growth hormone also declines with age and replacement with injections causes fairly dramatic changes. There is gain in strength, reversal of the muscle to fat ratio, and renewed sexual desire. HOWEVER, There is no evidence that hormone replacement of any type enhances longevity and many fears have been raised by such complications as blood clotting disorders and increased rates of some cancers.

OXIDATIVE STRESS THEORY

What a tempting theory of aging. Research is clear that oxidative stress increases with aging. It is also clear that certain oxidizing free radicals (e.g. superoxide, hydrogen peroxide, hydroxyl radical, etc.) are capable of damaging DNA. Many short term studies on mice and fruit flies support increased longevity when antioxidants are added to their diet. Some human studies also support the theory. Natural antioxidants are present on foods, especially fruits and vegetables. A list of foods rich in antioxidants can be found in an internet search. Despite this, the effect on longevity is controversial and there is little in long term human research to support supplemental antioxidant intake beyond the natural healthy diet high in fruits and vegetables. The strongest evidence in support of supplements are for Vitamin D (you can have your blood level checked), Omega 3 fatty acids, aspirin, and perhaps folic acid. Other than these, you may be wasting your money.

IS AGING NORMAL ?

Since it happens to all of us, though at different rates, can one call the process of aging "normal"? I prefer to define "normal" as expected changes with advancing age. What are they? Lets look at them system by system and consider those actions we can take to at least slow them down. I call it hanging onto our youth as long as possible.

Overall, you can expect to see decreased height, decreased weight, decreased body water content, increase in fat to lean body mass, increased wrinkling, and graying hair. Examine the details system by system and consider those actions we can take to protect these organs and delay this seemingly inevitable process.

1. Skin: The skin is the largest organ of our body. It's major functions include protecting us from the environment, cooling us when it is too hot and warming us when it is cold. This helps to keep our body temperature within very close tolerances. It provides a barrier to the invasion by bacteria. It minimizes damage from injury and abrasion. It blocks penetration of ultraviolet radiation and reduces Vitamin D produced but probably not enough to effect bone health or the prevention of some cancers. Ammonia and urea (toxic end products of metabolism) are excreted in sweat. Fine nerve endings in the skin convey touch, pain, heat, and cold. The rich blood supply can increase and decrease rapidly to aid in cooling

or can decrease shunting blood to internal organs when exposed to cold.

Because it is so visible we can watch the aging process. Note how your skin becomes thinner, so thin that you can see the blood vessels beneath the skin. It becomes very fragile and can tear and show bruising as the result of minor trauma due to capillary fragility. The sweat glands atrophy (shrink) making us more sensitive to heat, as the main mechanism for cooling is sweating and evaporation. Hair may thin in some areas and grow in others like in the ears and nose.

What can we do to protect this very vital organ? First of all is cleanliness. Wash away the harmful bacteria and the dead cells from the surface. Not only does this protect the skin but it is from these bacteria that we spread infectious diseases to ourselves and others. Minimize ultraviolet ray exposure by wearing long sleeved clothing of light color, hats with wide brims, and use sunblock creams of high number. This can be so effective that you may need to take supplemental vitamin D. It is worth having your level checked by a simple blood test. Wide variations in weight may damage the elastic fibers in the dermis, resulting in stretch marks called striae. In dry climates or in homes with heating or air conditioning, the skin can become dry and flaky. This is easily corrected with moisturizing creams. With proper care the skin can retain a youthful appearance and deadly cancers can be avoided.

2. Cardiovascular: Most of the changes that occur in our blood vessels are invisible to the naked eye. You may note the elongation and tortuousity which is apparent in superficial arteries. Perhaps the best place to see this in your temples. Inside the arteries there are more subtle changes going on. The innermost lining of the vessels is called the intima and it is slowly thickening. There is scarring in the middle layer (media) and the heart valves are thickening with scar tissue. But far more important are the changes that occur due to fatty substances in the blood. We have known about the harmful effects of cholesterol for many decades and focused upon diet as the best way to control the level. As important as diet is, it accounts for only about one fourth of the total. The remaining three fourths is synthesized in our liver and intestines. What can we do about that? First, understand there are different types of blood lipids. HDL, or high density lipoproteins, are GOOD cholesterols since they actually protect the blood vessels. The higher the proportion of the total cholesterol that is HDL, the better. LDL or low density lipoproteins are BAD and the lower the density, the worse it is. A third type is called triglycerides, also harmful and requiring different dietary restriction. The level all of these can be changed with proper diet and exercise. Fat levels in the diet should not exceed 20% and even lower is better. Carbohydrates (sugars and starches) contribute to the triglyceride level and

should be restricted as well. The ultimate goal of diet is to take in slightly fewer calories than you burn, a situation called UNDERNUTRITION. This differs from malnutrition since the former is a well balanced diet of low caloric value while the latter is unbalanced and of variable caloric value. At the same time one must exercise regularly. People often tell me that they work very hard and feel that is equivalent to exercise. Not true. One must commit to a period of time not less than 20 to 30 minutes of continuous exercise that is not interrupted by other activities. Your physician can calculate the exact amount and type of exercise most suitable for your health. When diet and exercise fail to reach the target levels of lipids in your blood, several medications can, singly or in combination, reach those values. The long term effect is dramatic in slowing, preventing or even reversing damage that has been done to the blood vessels and has been proven to reduce the risk of heart disease and stroke. Know your blood lipid levels and do whatever it takes to bring them in line. It is definitely worth the effort.

3. Kidneys: The kidneys contain over 600,000 tiny filters called glomeruli. These filters remove the waste chemical from the blood and retain the "good" chemicals to maintain chemical balance. That number gradually decreases as we age. Fortunately we start out with more than twice the number we need to maintain health and one

kidney can do the job. The chemical composition of our blood remains normal until very advanced age. The kidneys function optimally when there is adequate intake of water. Minimum intake should approach 6 to 8 glasses a day and increases with exposure to high temperatures and high humidity. Many medications are excreted through the kidneys, so close monitoring is required when drugs of this type are prescribed. To avoid toxicity, blood levels of the medication may be needed. Blood sugar levels must be controlled if you are diabetic and a protective medication called an ACE inhibitor or receptor blocker may be needed. Prevent kidney stones if you have a disorder that makes you prone to them. Promptly treat a kidney or other urinary tract infection. High blood pressure is especially damaging and must be controlled.

4. Lungs: The lungs are very elastic and little effort is required to expand them in normal breathing. That elasticity begins to decline after age 20 but may not be noticeable for many more years. The elasticity is about half at age 70 compared to age 20. The tiny hair cells (cilia) on the surface lining of the airways that constantly wave to move mucus and inhaled foreign materials and even bacteria and viruses out of the airways show decreased function, much like a worn toothbrush. Thus we are more susceptible to infections and must cough more to remove these substances. Air quality is of

foremost importance to lung function and has a major impact upon lung aging. Particulate matter, bacteria, viruses, and chemicals, either as gasses or mists, can produce lasting damage. Smoking is so terribly damaging that it is considered the number one cause of preventable illness and death. Even secondary smoke increases the risk of serious disease.

5. Eyes: Changes in near vision are often one of the first signs that we are aware of in the aging process. Print that used to be easy to read must be held further from the eyes to bring it into sharp focus. Most of us start out with "drugstore readers" which magnify and temporarily correct the problem. By this time everyone should have a thorough evaluation by an ophthalmologist to rule out more complex lens requirements and to detect early signs of avoidable problems. Of course, safety lenses should be worn whenever one is working with tools which produce dust or particulate matter. Ultraviolet light is harmful to the lens and retina. Eye shading hats or caps and glasses with UV protection should be worn whenever outside. Regular checkups, at least annually, are needed to diagnose vision damaging glaucoma (high pressure within the eye).

6. Hearing: This also decreases slowly and high frequencies are the first to go. Since most conversation takes place at lower frequencies

it may not be noticeable. However, background noise causes decreased ability to distinguish sounds. This is especially true if one has been exposed to loud noises such as power equipment, guns, jet engines and even loud music. Balance also decreases due to changes in the tiny hair cells in the inner ear. Hearing is essential to recognize many dangers. Imagine not being able to hear an oncoming vehicle or a call to "watch out." Protect your hearing with ear protectors for even brief exposure to high levels of noise. Play music softly. Treat ear infections promptly and thoroughly. Hearing can be improved in many ways, including hearing aids and surgical implants.

7. Taste becomes less sensitive and saliva may diminish. Food is, therefore, less appealing but can be enhanced with spices and creamy sauces. Food becomes less desirable and often there is weight loss. The diet may lack balance and consideration should be given to supplemental vitamins. It has been my practice to advise purchasing the cheapest brand of a multivitamin that is labeled as one per day. There may be special circumstances where your physician would advise a larger dose of a specific vitamin such as Vitamin D, but large doses called mega doses are probably a waste of money.

8. Smell: The sense of smell decreases and stronger stimuli are needed to be able to differentiate

between different smells. This can also affect the appreciation of food aromas and further lessen the desire for food. It can be dangerous if one cannot recognize the odor of escaping gas or dangerous chemicals.

9. Blood vessels: Arteries become somewhat stiffer with the result that the systolic blood pressure (the pressure when the heart contracts) tends to rise. Lengthening also occurs and can be seen where arteries are close to the skin as in the temple area. Because of the lengthening, the arteries become tortuous instead of lining up straight. Fatty deposits accumulate in the inner layer or endothelium. This is extremely important and is discussed in greater detail in the section on heart disease.

10. Urinary bladder: The bladder becomes more sensitive to the pressure of accumulated urine and we tend to relieve ourselves more frequently of smaller volumes. The stream becomes weaker and emptying may not be complete. There may increased urgency. Though these symptoms seem to occur in almost everyone, they may also be symptoms of disease. In women, childbirth may lead to relaxation of the pelvic floor. In men they may be signs of prostate enlargement or even cancer. They are more than just an annoyance when they interfere with restful sleep. Sleep deprivation has significant systemic effects.

Heart disease, obesity, and depression may be aggravated. It is also believed to weaken the immune system, making one more susceptible to disease.

11. Body fat: In early years we add fat, mostly beneath the skin. In later years we may lose body fat but what remains is mostly deep and around the inner organs. This type of deposition is associated with an increased risk of heart attacks and stroke and makes weight loss more urgent.

12. Bones: Bone is a living tissue. In youth, we build bone and bone strength increases in response to stress (exercise). In later years, bone density and strength gradually decline and we become more susceptible to fractures. Adequate intake of calcium (approximately 1000 milligrams per day but higher in postmenopausal women) combined with Vitamin D is essential. Blood level should be checked to determine individual status. Exercise stimulates the building of strong bone.

13. The connections between neurons (synapses) gradually decrease in number and changes occur in the chemical balance and microcirculation. This causes the so-called "senior moments," more scientifically described as normal age related memory lapses. Brain cells diminish in amazing numbers and the actual amount of "grey matter" decreases. As the brain loses cells, so does the

spinal cord. Reflexes are slowed and pose a special risk when driving or operating power equipment. Balance and coordination are impaired. The good news is that the brain can be stimulated by continued exercise and that one can actually grow new brain cells and activate pathways which have become inactive. Good mental exercise includes such activities as learning a new language, playing thought provoking games such as bridge, crossword puzzles, sudoku, or even writing a memoir. Statin drugs may delay the onset of Alzheimer's disease but more research is needed before this can become a standard recommendation.

14. Metabolism: The active thyroid hormone tends to decrease with age. This is frequently subclinical and must be detected by a simple blood test (TSH). Diet and exercise combined with hormone replacement usually control the symptoms and may reduce the incidence of heart disease.

15. Muscles: Muscle mass decreases with age but exercise against   resistance will reverse much of this loss and should be a part of everyone's daily program. There has been much interest in injections of human growth hormone which does, indeed, increase muscle mass and strength. There has been too little long-term study of this practice to assure that it does not have risks of major side effects.

16. Sexual changes: The sudden drop in hormone levels which women undergo during menopause can result in many uncomfortable symptoms. Physical changes also include decreased vaginal lubrication, shrinkage of the vaginal lining, and accelerated bone loss. The standard therapy for decades has been hormone replacement with either natural or synthetic hormones, identical to those formed by the woman's own ovaries. In recent years several fears have been raised over whether this treatment is appropriate. Studies showing increased incidences of breast cancers and blood coagulation problems have raised warnings about their use. In men, the decrease in hormone levels is gradual. Nevertheless, hormone therapy with testosterone or human growth hormone has been used to reduce the loss of muscle and bone mass and increase libido. Risks of long term side effects have limited their use.

17. Emotional changes. Feelings of depression, isolation, dependency can often be overcome by active social engagement. Continuing to work in one's occupation or profession or when this is not possible, volunteering in a charitable endeavor. Service clubs, church groups, and social clubs all offer continued outlets for engagement. Travel offers new opportunities.

All of these are so common as we age and are seemingly not associated with any known disease process that I consider them to be expected changes, part of a normal process or perhaps better referred to as a usual change.

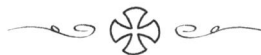

WHAT ELSE SHORTENS OUR LIVES ?

LIFESTYLE CHOICES

A sk any insurance company what lifestyle choices shorten your life expectancy. They have mountains of statistics carefully evaluated by numbers crunchers called actuaries. They must be accurate in their predictions because their financial risk is increased if you engage in or participate in these activities. Most insurers will rate you, meaning charge a higher premium, if you smoke, drink alcoholic beverages to excess, or if you are significantly overweight. Also, you may be rated if you use drugs, even prescribed medication, or are exposed to radiation. Some will increase your rate if you are in a stressful occupation or one that exposes you to harmful chemicals or gasses. See the partial list below of things that carry a significant risk of shortening your life.

Aviation
Base-jumping
Bungee jumping

Hang gliding
Hot air ballooning
Rock climbing or mountaineering
Scuba diving
Skiing
Skydiving
Surfing
White water rafting
Motorcycling
Firefighting
Police work
Mining

That is not a complete list and insurers vary in what activities they consider hazardous enough to raise premiums, but you can see how you can avoid many things to help increase your own longevity.

YOUR OCCUPATION

See in the chart on the next page how great an effect your choice of occupation may have upon your expected longevity. These statistics were collected and published by the United States Department of Labor and reflect the experience in 2010, the latest available at this time.

Number and rate of fatal occupational injuries, by major civilian occupation group, 2010*

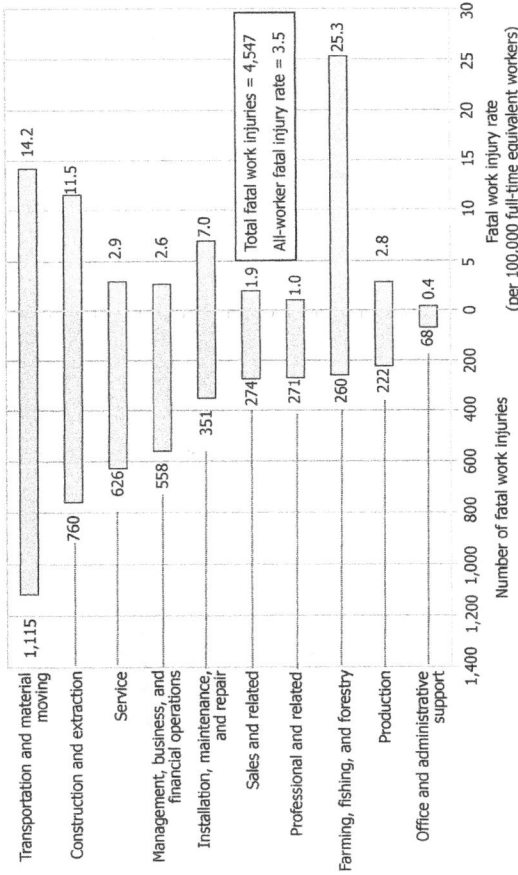

Occupation group	Number of fatal work injuries	Fatal work injury rate
Transportation and material moving	1,115	14.2
Construction and extraction	760	11.5
Service	626	2.9
Management, business, and financial operations	558	2.6
Installation, maintenance, and repair	351	7.0
Sales and related	274	1.9
Professional and related	271	1.0
Farming, fishing, and forestry	260	25.3
Production	222	2.8
Office and administrative support	68	0.4

Total fatal work injuries = 4,547
All-worker fatal injury rate = 3.5

Number of fatal work injuries

Fatal work injury rate
(per 100,000 full-time equivalent workers)

Although transportation and material moving occupations had the highest number of fatal work injuries in 2010, the highest fatal work injury rate among major occupational groups was for farming, fishing, and forestry occupations.

*Data for 2010 are preliminary.
NOTE: Fatal injury rates exclude workers under the age of 16 years, volunteers, and resident military. The number of fatal work injuries represents total published fatal injuries before the exclusions. For additional information on the fatal work injury rate methodology changes please see http://www.bls.gov/iif/oshnotice10.htm.
SOURCE: U.S. Bureau of Labor Statistics, U.S. Department of Labor, 2011.

WHERE YOU LIVE

When you examine life expectancy at birth by country of residence you may be surprised. The latest numbers published by the government show the little principality of Monaco has the longest at 89.73 years and the shortest in Angola at 38.76 years. The United States ranks 50th at 78.37 years. These numbers can be very misleading as so many factors are at play besides the country itself. For example, Japan ranks 5th at 82.25 years yet Japanese living in the United States have the same expectancy that they would have if they lived in Japan. These numbers are a mixture of racial, ethnic, cultural, and social differences that have a greater influence than the country itself. In Ireland, for example there are two cities only eight miles apart (Calton and Lenzie), where the longevity differs by 28 years between the two. One is a very poor area and the other a wealthy area. Guess which one has the longer life span. Of course, the wealthy neighborhood wins. Social status has an immense effect.

TOXINS

The list of environmental toxins is so comprehensive, there is no way to address it fully in this section. You cannot turn on your television set without being bombarded with ads soliciting your involvement with class action lawsuits regarding exposure to asbestos or medications which have been shown to have adverse side effects. There are many occupational exposures to dusts, chemicals or fumes, all regulated by the Environmental Protection Agency. Of direct concern to all of us is the presence of toxic substances in the food supply. Such things as pesticides, herbicides and fungicides are used on crops to increase production. Traces of these chemicals have been shown in experimental conditions to cause cancer and neurologic disease. Despite this evidence, there is no direct human evidence to confirm a relationship to the diseases. Many, however, welcome the availability of organic food alternatives to eliminate what they believe to be an unnecessary exposure. Public water supplies are monitored regularly to keep levels of heavy metals and other chemicals below what is considered safe amounts. Plastics are another area of concern. How would we get along without them? Yet many have been shown to release small amounts of phthalates which have been shown in the laboratory to increase cancers. Lead based paint is not used in this country but products from other countries may still have it, an especial risk to children. Meanwhile, what can you do? Stay away from cigarette smoke, breathe the freshest air you can (in-home air filtration), and wash fresh fruits and vegetables. When possible, avoid prepared foods.

RADIATION

You cannot escape some harmful radiation. The sun's ultraviolet rays, very insidiously, do major cumulative harm to the skin. The damage ranges from a dry scaly thickening called actinic keratosis (precancerous), to basal cell cancer, squamous cell cancer and the most aggressive form called melanoma. You have control over this exposure by using sunblock creams, wearing wide-brimmed hats and long-sleeved light color clothing.

The most common form of penetrating radiation is radon within the home. This can be readily tested for with available kits and corrective action can be undertaken if the levels are high. Then there is background radiation, that which comes from traces of radioactive material in the soil. Cosmic radiation, which comes from the sun, is greater in high elevations where there is less filtration by the atmosphere. There is a small amount (about 11%) that comes from within our own bodies. Radioactive elements are deposited in bones and certain tissues and continue to radiate. Nuclear fallout from bomb testing and accidents in nuclear energy plants are another source. The recent accident in Japan following the earthquake and tsunami left dangerous levels for several miles. Fears that dangerous levels would reach the United States were unfounded as the dilution in the atmosphere left very low levels. The area where we have the greatest control is medical procedures. A simple chest x-ray gives a tiny dose of radiation, but more complex procedures such as scans, fluoroscopic tests, and cancer treatments give significant exposure. Be sure the procedures are truly necessary. Remember that all radiation is cumulative so all of these need to be added together to determine if you have a real risk.

Finally, smoking and other tobacco use almost double the risk.

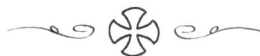

.

PERSONAL CHOICES

SMOKING TOBACCO is the number one cause of preventable premature death and disability in the United States and probably the world. Smokers need to face the fact that it is not just a habit but a serious drug addiction which leads to disease and death. There are far more deaths and serious consequences from nicotine than from hard drugs such as cocaine, heroin or meth. In fact, cocaine addicts will frequently admit that it is harder to quit nicotine than cocaine.

Alcoholic beverages rival nicotine as an addictive drug with serious consequences. Most fatal automobile accidents are alcohol related. It takes so little to alter ones reflexes and judgment and the drinker seems to be the last one to recognize that there is a problem. I wonder how many injuries working around machinery, or falls in the home are precipitated by alcohol. Certainly crime and violence are directly related to excessive use of alcohol. There is a paradox, however, as small amounts of alcohol seem to slightly improve longevity. Some research points to red wine as the most beneficial in small sensible amounts.

When we think of deaths due to drugs, we usually think first of illegal narcotics, but that is only a small part of the picture. Far more deaths are caused by prescription and over the counter medicines than illegal drugs. Even when an approved drug is prescribed for the appropriate cause and in the proper dose, serious risks occur. It could be an unexpected allergic reaction, a known but rare side effect, a previously unknown idiosyncrasy or a cross reaction with another medicine you are taking. That does not mean that you should not take medicine when prescribed but be aware of the "risk-reward" and don't take medicine for minor symptoms or without due consideration. Be sure your doctor knows all medicines you are taking, including over the counter and supplemental products. It is best to get all your medicines from the same pharmacist and ask him about possible interactions and warnings.

MEDICAL CONDITIONS

Of the thousands of diseases or illnesses that can result in premature death, I want to focus on the ten most common causes of death in those over 65 and suggest how to prevent or manage them. The numbers come from the Center for Disease Control/ NationalCenter for Health Statistics last updated in February 2011.

HEART DISEASE

Heart disease remains number one by a pretty wide margin and you can have a major influence on its development by your actions. There are many types of heart disease over which you have little control except through early diagnosis and treatment, so regular check-ups and tests are encouraged. Not smoking is of extreme importance and yes, you can quit. Sometimes it is hard and you may need medical and group support but it is worth it a thousand times over. Do it!!! It is a killer addiction. Coronary vascular disease is the most frequent type and much of it is undiagnosed because it may not cause symptoms until right before sudden death. Lipids (fats) are the main culprits but it is more complex than you might think. There are HDLs (high density lipoproteins) which are good cholesterols as they actually protect the blood vessels. LDLs (low density lipoproteins) are the bad ones, and the lower the density the worse they are. Triglycerides are another lipid which comes not only from fats but also from carbohydrates. The level of each can easily be measured by a blood test. Sometimes abnormal levels can be corrected by proper diet and exercise. When that is not enough, there are several proven medicines that, in the right dosage and combination, can result in normal levels. This will not only protect the blood vessels from deposits called plaques, but, if the levels are low enough, can actually remove existing deposits.

These plaques start very early in life and progress silently and slowly over the years. When they get big enough, they block the flow of blood to the heart muscle (heart attack or "coronary".) Check your levels early in life and at intervals as you age and take action before the vessels are destroyed. Hypertension and diabetes both accelerate the process and both can be controlled. Diagnose them early by checkups, especially if they exist in other members of your family. Each one is improved by diet and exercise.

If an artery becomes completely blocked by an aggregation of platelets or a clot, the result may be a "heart attack" if the offending artery is a coronary artery or a stroke if the artery supplies the brain. Hypertension (elevated blood pressure), by itself, produces damage to both the heart and blood vessels and accelerates the damage caused by elevated cholesterol. There has long been controversy over what level of pressure constitutes hypertension. The general rule is that the lower levels are associated with less disease than the higher levels. Almost all physicians agree that systolic blood pressure (when the heart is contracting) above 140 millimeters of mercury and/or a diastolic pressure (when the heart is between beats) over 85 millimeters of mercury are points when at least the first steps of treatment should be considered. These first steps are weight reduction, reduced salt intake, and regular aerobic exercise. The decision to start medicine for control is far more complex and must be answered by your physician considering many factors besides the level of pressure alone. Control of blood lipids is essential and should be initiated as soon as elevation is discovered and continued throughout life. Weight control, diet and exercise may be enough but frequently medication is required to reach the target levels. Doctors' supervision and monitoring is needed to determine dosage side effects and whether a combination of drugs is needed. Control of hypertension and blood lipid levels can add many years to your life. Modern surgical techniques including clot dissolution during cardiac catheterization, placement of stents, and bypass surgery add many years to ones life despite advanced arterial disease.

CANCER

2. You may be surprised at how much you can do to prevent, cure or control many cancers. Cancer has become the number two killer of our time. It takes many forms and has many names, usually related to the organ affected. The underlying principle is that cells grow without the usual controls on growth rate and replace the normal cells. These cancer cells usually do not function and crowd out the functioning cells and may spread to other organs. As this process continues, the outcome is death. Great advances have been made in understanding the causes of cancer and in developing treatments that influence the pattern of growth. Some can be cured, especially

if discovered early before it has had time to spread. The real advance has been in understanding the causes. There isn't just one cause but many different causes of different types of cancer. The list is long but I will mention a few examples. Asbestos dust is a cause of lung cancer and cancer of the pleura (lining of the lung). Levels of exposure once thought to be safe are now known to be toxic. Inhaling fumes from or skin contact with benzene can lead to leukemia or lymphoma. The viruses which cause hepatitis B or C have each been linked to cancer of the liver. There is a long list of food additives that have been banned because of a link to cancers. As we learn more about what causes cancers we can do more to prevent them. The BIG ONE, however, is SMOKING. It is the number one cause of preventable cancers, and not just of the lungs but many cancers, even in distant parts of the body. Prevention is far more effective than treatment.

STROKE

3. Stroke is another form of vascular disease but, in this case, the target organ is the brain. Damage to the blood vessels leading to the brain is the same as described above for heart disease (blood lipids, high blood pressure and diabetes). If the blood vessel that is blocked is a small one, there may be just a momentary speech impediment, numbness, dizzy spell, confusion, trouble seeing clearly, or maybe a

severe headache. This may clear up in a few minutes but must not be disregarded. It is a warning sign of worse to come. The technical term for these episodes is "Transient Ischemic Attacks". If a larger blood vessel is blocked it may cause paralysis of one side of the body, inability to speak, and may progress to coma. Usually there is permanent loss of function but great strides have been made in rehabilitation and treatment. If there is immediate intervention, the residual effects may be minimized. Call 911 and get to the ER immediately. If the blockage is in the main artery to the brain (carotid), which is in the neck, it may be corrected with surgery or stenting. Again, prevention is better than treatment. Discover blood lipid problems early in life and correct them, control blood pressure and, if diabetic, control blood sugar.

CHRONIC OBSTRUCTIVE PULMONARY DISEASE (COPD)

4. Chronic Obstructive Pulmonary Disease is the fourth leading cause of death and a major cause of long-term disability. If you could see, under the microscope, how very fragile the walls of the tiny air sacs (alveoli) are you could understand how sensitive they are to anything but clean air. COPD is almost completely preventable. Smoke, noxious gasses, chemical fumes and dusts are all very harmful and some can cause permanent damage. But, by far,

the most common cause is inhalation of tobacco smoke either as the smoker or being nearby (second hand smoke), and the damage is cumulative. Every cigarette adds further damage and the change is so insidious that it is not apparent sometimes for years. By then, the damage may not be reversible. Do not use tobacco products, live in air-polluted locations or engage in occupations that expose you to "bad" air.

PNEUMONIA

5. Pneumonia is an infection or inflammation deep within the lungs (alveoli) usually caused by either viral or bacterial infection, occasionally fungal, and rarely caused by parasites or toxic exposure. Because it involves the alveoli, where the exchange of oxygen and carbon dioxide occur, it interferes with respiration and can be fatal. Previous damage to the bronchi by such things as smoke inhalation or infections increases the likelihood of pneumonia. Immunization to the viruses of influenza and the bacteria pneumococcus greatly reduces risk and should be maintained for influenza annually and to pneumococcus at approximately ten-year intervals. Simple hand washing prevents many cases. When pneumonia happens in the hospital environment it may be particularly serious as many antibiotic resistant bacteria live in that atmosphere and can be quickly spread. Medicines and diseases that interfere

with immunity make one especially at risk. Another serious type is aspiration pneumonia. Especially in the elderly or patients with concurrent diseases, swallowing may be weakened and food can enter the respiratory tract. Disease such as reflux or anything associated with vomiting may be responsible. The infection which results is due to multiple bacteria of the intestinal tract and may be very resistant to the usual antibiotics. The death rate is high for this type of pneumonia.

DIABETES

6. Almost everyone knows the relationship between sugar and diabetes, but it is a far more complex problem than just that. First of all, there are three types. Type 1 often comes on in youth but can occur at any age. Its cause is not fully understood but most believe that it is an autoimmune disease perhaps set off by a viral infection. Our own immune system destroys the insulin producing cells of the pancreas leaving one dependent on insulin injections. Type 2 is quite different. It is genetic and that gene is "turned on" by factors such as improper diet and excessive weight. The insulin secreting cells can be stimulated by medicines to produce more but there is strong resistance to the insulin and supplemental injections are frequently required. Even then, unless there are strict controls on dietary intake of foods that contain carbohydrates that are digested to simple sugar, safe

levels of blood sugar are not possible. The epidemic of obesity that is so widespread now has caused a major increase in the incidence of diabetes. Sadly the symptoms are so vague that the disease is often not discovered for years until complications are already present. Symptoms may include excessive thirst, excessive urination and unexplained weight loss. A third type is called gestational diabetes, meaning that it occurs during pregnancy and goes away after delivery. It is usually easy to control and it is routine to test for it when pregnancy occurs. The risk of developing type 2 diabetes is fairly high for about five years after delivery. Some physicians use the term pre-diabetes for those patients whose blood sugar is above the levels called normal but not high enough to make a certain diagnosis. Whether this is a special type or not, it certainly is a warning to maintain a proper diet and recheck blood sugar levels, at least once a year.

Discovering diabetes early and instituting control measures that include diet, exercise and medication is of paramount importance because the complications of diabetes are disastrous. The small blood vessels are damaged leading to blindness, kidney failure, amputations and higher risk of heart attacks and strokes. Longevity is reduced by an average of 10 years. Don't wait for symptoms to be obvious: check regularly, at least annually and even more frequently if you have a family history or predisposing condition.

ACCIDENTS

7. "Accident don't just happen, there is always a cause." That is a quote from my mother. If there is a cause then there is a preventive action.

Look at automobile accidents. Fatalities reached a high of 45,836 in 2005 and the good news is that there has been a steady reduction to 37,261 in 2008. This is more related to safety features on automobiles than to greater responsibility on the part of drivers. Factors contributing to the fatalities are alcohol, distraction, and speeding which account for about 70% of the total. Those are all things we can modify by our own actions.

Other types of accidents I prefer to call unintentional injuries. In 2008 the National Hospital Ambulatory Medical Care Survey reported that there were 28.4 million emergency department visits for unintentional injuries. I'll bet there were many more that that treated at home.

In the same survey, 123,706 were fatal. There were 22,632 deaths due to falls and 29,846 due to poisoning. Many of these can be avoided by such simple tasks as driving defensively, accident proofing the home with grab rails in slippery areas such as the tub and shower, avoiding use of throw rugs, putting poisonous items in a locked cabinet out of reach of inquisitive children and using extra caution when using sharp tools.

SEPTICEMIA

8. Septicemia is often known as blood poisoning. Despite all of our advances in preventing and treating infections, some are still overwhelming and enter the blood stream where it can destroy organs throughout the body. A simple cut or skin abrasion can be the entry point of the bacteria. Having one's teeth cleaned can inject bacteria into the blood stream. Septicemia is most likely to occur in a patient following surgery, trauma, or during treatment for a concurrent illness. Medicines such as chemotherapy will increase susceptibility. Treatment is difficult because many organisms may be involved and major organs may fail before the infection can be controlled. There is a high mortality. Antibiotics may be given prophylactically in high-risk surgery. Even minor skin infections should be carefully cleansed and treated with local triple antibiotic ointment and covered with a bandage.

NEPHRITIS

9. Nephritis is an inflammation of the kidneys. It can be due to bacterial infection but more frequently is part of autoimmune disorders that affect other organs of the body. Lupus is a prime example of a systemic disease in which nephritis may play an important role. All causes of nephritis interfere with elimination of waste products and may result

in uremia (renal failure). Many medications must be eliminated in the urine and even mildly reduced renal function can result in toxic blood levels despite what would be the usual dose of the substance. The most common cause of renal failure is diabetes.

ALZHEIMER'S DISEASE

10. Four genes have been discovered which are related to Alzheimer's disease. Most commonly the disease has a late onset, meaning that the clinical manifestations of the disease are likely to occur after age 60 and progress slowly. The other form, early onset, may occur well before the age of 60 and progresses more rapidly. This form is clearly genetic. It is less clear what part genetics play in the late onset type. The diagnosis can only be made with certainty by examining brain tissue. Other forms of dementia such as multiple small strokes may mimic Alzheimer's. Environmental factors seem to influence the rate of progression or delay the onset. Physical exercise and mental exercise, such as learning a new language or playing card games that require solving problems or memory, seem to have a protective effect. Differentiating between normal aging changes and those related to Altzheimer's may be difficult in the early stages. Getting lost on a familiar route may signal the onset. Personality change, loss of interest, misplacing common items, forgetting names of family members, and language difficulty

are the more common signs. Medications have been developed with minor but ultimately disappointing benefits. The most one can do to prevent the onset of the disease is to remain physically active, participate in challenging activities and remain socially active. Omega 3 fatty acids, antioxidants, statins, and non-steroidal anti-inflammatory drugs have all been proposed as preventatives, but solid evidence of their effectiveness is lacking. A vaccine is being studied but is not yet ready for clinical use.

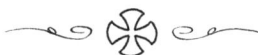

REACH YOUR POTENTIAL

A lot of things must come together to reach your individual potential. Genes can only set the stage. It is the environment that will cut short that potential.

The Administration on Aging is an agency of the U.S. Department of Health and Human Services. It attributes the dramatic increase in the aging population to "advances in science, technology, and medicine leading to reductions in infant and maternal mortality, infectious and parasitic diseases, occupational safety measures, and improvements in nutrition and education." That is certainly true when applied to whole populations. However, I want to focus on the enormous influence you can have on your own personal longevity. No new scientific breakthroughs are needed to reach the goal of 120 years if one starts soon enough. Ideally our children should be brought up understanding the choices they must make in their lives to achieve good health and longevity. However, it is never too late to start. Even in the senior years, changing lifestyle and following the principles outlined in the foregoing chapters will add years to ones lifespan.

LETS GET DOWN TO BUSINESS
WHAT SHALL I DO NOW?

1. Don't ever use tobacco products. If you have already started, QUIT NOW and get whatever help you can to break this terrible addiction. Help your close family members and associates to quit as well since their second hand smoke puts you at risk too. It is the number one cause of preventable disease.

2. Follow the proper diet. It should focus on vegetables and fruits. Lean meat servings should not be larger than your cell phone. Quantities should be limited so that your body is as fat free as possible. The term undernutrition has been suggested to describe a balanced diet of total caloric value slightly less than your body needs. This very slight starvation seems to turn on vital body defenses and lengthens life.

3. Exercise is vital. For some, this means joining a gym or fitness center and participating in group activities. Special equipment is not needed. It is fine, but not necessary if you can discipline yourself to a regular routine. Just walking 20-30 minutes a day is enough combined with simple muscle resistance exercises. It can be done at home. My favorite is swimming. It is aerobic and the water provides the resistance, yet there is no weight or strain on joints.

4. Get enough education to assure that you will have a good job with economic security. It should be a something you can enjoy doing your whole life. Stress is greatly reduced when you are having fun and people with above average means live longer.

5. Pick a place to live and work where there is clean air. Be sure there are good medical facilities nearby and that you have established a strong relationship with a personal physician. Have regular checkups and follow through on any clues that suggest an underlying disease or susceptibility to a disease. In today's environment, a group practice may offer the best alternative to an individual practitioner as they are becoming harder and harder to find. If you have a medical problem, learn all you can about it and become a knowledgeable partner with your doctor. Genome studies which will reveal susceptibility to conditions or diseases have just been made available and in many cases you will be able to take action to prevent or delay expression of that gene.

6. Get every immunization available and indicated for you (age and sex influence the decision). Keep them up to date. At this time, there is NO credible evidence that immunizations cause disease, and much research has been done to verify this.

7. Make wise lifestyle decisions. The momentary thrill of certain activities is certainly not worth the risks involved. It is not much to give up when the price could be lifelong disability or death. Make your goal to reach 120 years.

8. Keep exercising your mind by reading, studying, and traveling to new places. Learn a new language. Write a life history. Play challenging mind games such as bridge or Sudoku. Don't retire unless you replace that occupation with another or expand your hobby interests.

9. Remain socially active with group activities within your church, service club, professional organization or other interest group. The greatest satisfaction will come from those activities where you are using your talents and skills to serve others.

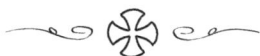

LOVE EVERY MINUTE

This book promised you more than how to achieve increased longevity. Yes, it has shown you the ways in which you can delay aging and even turn off "bad genes" (those which would make you susceptible to diseases or conditions which could shorten your life). If you read those words expecting to escape the aging process described in previous chapters or escape the diseases, accidents or circumstances that shorten our lives, you misread my intention. They only set the stage and show a very rewarding path in terms of longevity. You will still face heartaches, diseases, injuries, and accidents, perhaps with residual physical impairments. You may fall short of your planned goals in business or personal relationships. You may fail in many ways. You will suffer many of the same challenges that every one else must face. Would you still want longer life? Some of you will fear the ravages you have seen in other folks. The key is how you will cope with these obstacles. Can you be happy and optimistic despite these defeats?

The Declaration of Independence assures us that one of our inalienable rights is the "pursuit of happiness". Note carefully that it says pursuit without any guarantees that we can accomplish that goal. So, what is it that makes us happy?

The late great comedian Groucho Marx said "Each morning when I open my eyes I say to myself: I, not events, have the power to make me happy or unhappy today. I can choose which it shall be. Yesterday is dead, tomorrow hasn't arrived yet. I have just one day, today, and I'm going to be happy in it." Do we really have that much influence or control upon our happiness? Yes we do!

Well then, what are we going to pursue today to make ourselves happy? For many, it is reaching the top in their profession or occupation. There is a feeling of accomplishment and power in recognition or even fame which gives us a sense of importance. That feels good. Along with that there is usually increased income, even riches. Now we can buy those things that give us pleasure. But accomplishments, riches and fame give us pleasure that is not synonymous with happiness. Also it tends to be transient and shallow. Just look at the number of entertainment idols, athletes, and political leaders who seem to have everything, yet they succumb to alcohol and drugs to diminish their pain. This goes far beyond these pursuits. Well then, if not fame, wealth, power and sex, what should we look for in our pursuit of happiness? What will give us the strength to overcome adversity?

Many would argue, myself included, that length of life may not even be the most important thing. So far this book has completely ignored the other YOU.

I believe there is far more to YOU than a miraculously organized combination of chemicals. What is it that makes us so special? It is the quality that makes each of us so different. Our bodies and our DNA are amazingly similar but our spirit, soul and our personalities are very different. They are as important to each of us as our body and are, in fact, the most important parts. If we were a boat or airplane, they would be our rudders. If we were rockets, they would be called our guidance system. We could not function without them. The direction that we follow in our life would be aimless and haphazard. The length of our lives is far less important than the quality of our life. What is our soul? Do we exercise any control over it?

If you feel that we are just a miraculously organized combination of chemicals that came together and took on their specialized functions by chance, just read on.

Our most remarkable body is made up of only a few dollars worth of chemicals. They are arranged in an even more remarkable way into interrelated functioning organs. Each cell has its own specialized function and relates to all the other cells and is a part of this whole that we call the human body. Some feel this all came about by chance with the essential chemicals coming together in a primordial mud or soup in the early days of our planet's existence forming the initial forms of life. Can you even imagine the odds against these chemicals coming together in the right concentrations, at the right temperature, for the appropriate length of time to form a living, reproducing organism which evolved into what we are today? If you said yes, let me ask you to look again at the basic structure of DNA and the precise location of all the atoms that make up its structure. DNA is the key to life and reproduction. Below is a depiction of a segment of DNA and beside it is a depiction of the chemical structure of just two of the proteins making up the base pairs that must be precisely aligned.

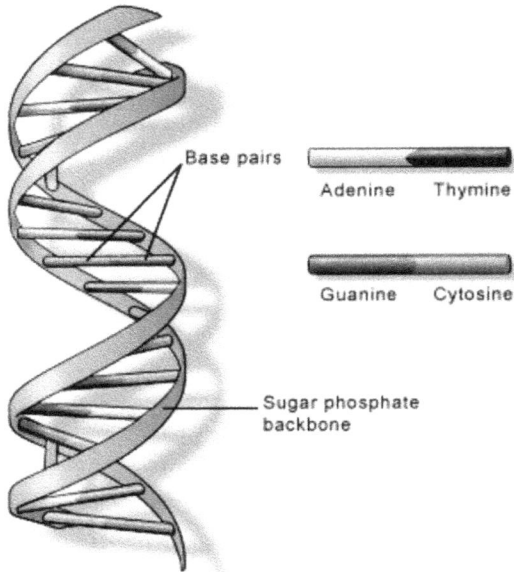

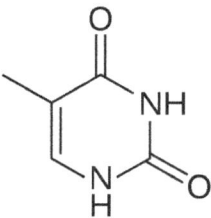

Thymine

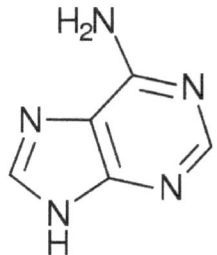

Adenine

Just try to calculate the odds again that they could all come together by chance. The odds are incomprehensible. Yes, I believe in intelligent design, intelligence far, far beyond human understanding. I also believe in evolution as an adaptation to the environment. But it cannot account for the multiplicity of species on this earth or the very special nature of the individual human being, man.

Is duration of life the most important thing? What about the quality of life? What about happiness despite the challenges we must face? Are we just a human-like robot? Is there a purpose to life? Is there a soul? Most importantly, is there a God?

Science, rather than disproving the existence of God, has piled up overwhelming evidence proving an intelligent design. If you think otherwise, I ask you, no, I beg you to read the free e-book by Tihomir Dimitrov titled 50 Nobel Laureates and Other Great Scientists Who believe in God. Everyone should read this excellent book. He lists the scientists by name and includes quotes from them on their beliefs. Think of some great scientists whom you respect and look to see if they are on the list. I'll bet many of them are. You can access it at http://nobelists.net. The author lists Nobel Writers of the 20th & 21st Centuries, Nobel Peace Laureates, Founders of Modern Science from the 16th century to the 21st century, and the great philosophers from the 17th to the 21st century. He also lists others and their beliefs about Jesus. If all of these great minds believe based upon solid evidence, shouldn't you also take heed?

MOVING EXAMPLES

My entire professional career of over 60 years has been in direct patient care. I think I had the finest medical education possible at Northwestern University but it is what I learned from my patients that truly enriched my life, revealed to me my purpose in life and strengthened my faith. I treated many patients with serious, life threatening and, in many cases, terminal illnesses where I was helpless to alter the course of their disease. It was in these instances that their courage and faith had its greatest impact upon me. Let me relate just two examples burned deeply into my memory

I'd like to tell the true story of a couple of patients whose approach to adversity profoundly affected me. How much I wish that I could have their strength.

In fact, one patient changed my whole attitude on disability. He was a young man who had suffered a fractured neck with spinal cord injury. He had no use of his legs and almost none in his arms and hands. A little movement in his fingers let him control a sophisticated electric wheel chair. He had to be fed, bathed and moved by others. Depressing? One would think so. However he always had a smile on his face when I visited and an incredibly optimistic outlook. He had strong support from his adoring wife and extended family. He was a Christian and reassured me that he had no fear of death. BUT the thing that hit me the hardest was the day I walked into his room to assess his progress in overcoming an infection, requiring intravenous antibiotics. He had been propped up into an almost sitting position with the over-the-bed table pulled up close to him. On it was a phone and he was engaged in a conversation he interrupted to talk to me. His wife punched in the phone numbers and a small earpiece and microphone were held in place on his head. I asked about it and he told me he held a telemarketing job to help support his family. I held back my tears until I was out of the room but then let go. Ever since that day, I do not like to use the term disabled, preferring to describe these things as impairments. Does an impairment cause disability or is it an inability to confront the impairment and adjust to it that leads to disability? Despite a severe impairment, this young man was able to focus upon what he had rather than what he did not have. His life was still rich with the love of his wife and family, more than enough to keep him happy. His Christian faith promised him even more and he was a true believer.

I have seen many patients with impairments who requested that I fill out forms needed to support a claim for benefits. A lot of them qualified using the standards set out by the insurance companies or governmental agencies and I complied. But I always remembered that paralyzed young man and thought how much better off these patients would have been if only they had accepted their circumstances and functioned to the maximum they were able.

The second case was also a young man in his mid 20's. I was asked by his primary physician to see him and to help diagnose what seemed to be a strange disease affecting both of his lungs. While I was taking his history, he recalled something he had not told the primary physician. He had travelled through a dust storm in Arizona on his way to Houston. This was exciting news to me as the changes on his chest X-ray were consistent with a fungal disease not too uncommon in the southwest called valley fever. Immediately I ordered the tests to verify that diagnosis and was surprised when they all came back negative. We decided that the only way to get a complete and accurate diagnosis was to do an open lung biopsy. A thoracic surgeon was called in to do this procedure. The next day we went to the pathology lab to view the biopsy slides with the pathologist. As soon as he focused on the slide he said, "Oh, this is bad news. It is cancer which has spread from another organ, probably from the pancreas or stomach." We all knew this was a death sentence as there was no treatment available at that time with a hope of cure, and probably no significant prolongation of life. Death seemed to be only weeks away. None of us wanted the task of delivering this news to the patient. I had a very good relationship with the patient and at the urging of the other physicians, I agreed to do it. I entered the room and indulged in a little small talk trying to think of the right words. When I finally got to the point and gave the bad news and the grim prognosis, he looked me directly in the eyes and, after a pause, he said, "At a time like this, it is great to be a Christian." I could not hold back the tears. I had never experienced such a strong faith in such a young person. He said that he had a good life and that he was ready to face whatever came. He was not depressed but was able to accept and adjust even to this grim prognosis.

These young men had found the way to happiness even in the face of terrible adversity. I believe that I have found that way in my own life.

Yes, I believe strongly in the soul. It is that other part of us that is indestructible and immortal. It is that quality which make us unique. Just yesterday I watched as a human-like robot was shown on television. The robot looked very real and as it talked and responded to questions it changed facial expressions and moved its lips in sync with the words. It will take very little refinement to fool us into believing that it is human. But no matter how well it can mimic our appearance it does not have this mystic quality that I call one's soul.

Was the source of their strength in the face of tremendous adversity some secret? NO. It is right in front of our face, yet we may spend a large part of our lives discovering it. Or, we may reject it because it is so incredible. It is all laid out in a book that has been the best seller every year since it was first published. Yes, I mean the Bible. In it, we were commanded to have "no other Gods before me." Too many people stumble on the word "God." What image comes to your mind as you consider who God is? As a child, I envisioned a big all-powerful person who looked like us and who lived in the clouds. After all, the Bible states that we were created in His image. Michelangelo's painting in the Sistine Chapel reinforced that perception with God's hand reaching down to his creation of man. No wonder so many deny God's existence. I have come to the conclusion that understanding the creator, or creative force, or cosmic force is beyond my comprehension and I accept the name God because my mind can handle that. We are unable to find the words in our language to describe with any accuracy such an incredible power. I believe in the Big Bang theory of the creation of the universe, but not as the atheists do. I think science is just delving deeper into the mechanism God used in creating the universe. Certainly it required a creator to power it and depends upon an incredible degree of intelligence.

If you still have a problem accepting such a higher power, then listen to the words of atheist Bertrand Russell found in Rick Warren's book The Purpose Driven Life, "Unless you assume a God, the question of life's purpose is meaningless." From your relationship with God, life becomes purposeful, rich and rewarding. I strongly recommend that you read The Purpose Driven Life. The chapter that impacted me the greatest is " What Matters Most." In it he states "Life is all about love."

LOVE

Long ago, in my struggle to try to understand God, I took to heart the words of the apostle John. "Everyone who loves is a child of God and knows God, but the unloving know nothing of God. For God is love, and his love was disclosed to us in this, that he sent his only Son into the world to bring us life." 1 John 4:8-10 (The New English Bible) Instead of trying to envision something superhuman, for the first time, I looked upon the spiritual being. It made everything much clearer to me. The driving force in this world is love and Jesus was love in human form. He lived a life in which all decisions were based upon love of one's neighbor. In such an environment great strength comes from such relationships. Not carnal love but rather the love described by the apostle Paul in his letter to the Corinthian church. 1 Corinthians 13, The New English Bible

"And now I will show you the best way of all. I may speak in tongues of men and angels, but if I am without love, I am a sounding gong or a clanging cymbal. I may have the gift of prophesy, and know every hidden truth; I may have faith strong enough to move mountains; but if I have no love, I am nothing. I may dole out all I possess, or even give my body to be burnt, but if I have no love, I am none the better. Love is patient; love is kind and envies no one. Love is never boastful, not conceited, nor rude; never selfish, not quick to take offense. Love keeps no score of wrongs; does not gloat over other men's sins, but delights in the truth. There is nothing love cannot face; there is no limit to its faith, its hope, its endurance. Love will never come to an end. Are there prophets? Their work will be over. Are there tongues of ecstasy? They will cease. Is there knowledge? It all will vanish away; for our knowledge and our prophesy alike are partial, and the partial vanishes when wholeness comes. When I was a child, my speech, my outlook, and my thoughts were all childish. When I grew up, I had finished with childish things. Now we see only puzzling reflections in a mirror, but then we shall see face to face. My knowledge now is partial; then it will be whole, like God's knowledge of me. In a word there are three things that last forever: faith, hope and love; but the greatest of them all is love."

A life filled with love will be a life of the greatest happiness and you will be able to cope with all life's challenges.

Now, what was the meaning of the secondary title to this book? It was not a statement of fact but, rather, a command. Spend your life with love (GOD) as your guide and you will look forward to each new day.

Time is too slow
For those who wait
Too swift for those who fear

Too short for those who rejoice

But for those who love, Time is Eternity

Henry Van Dyke

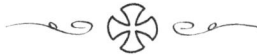

CITATION

www.ingramcontent.com/pod-product-compliance
Lightning Source LLC
Chambersburg PA
CBHW031006090426
42737CB00008B/701